SMOOTHIES FOR THYROID HEALING

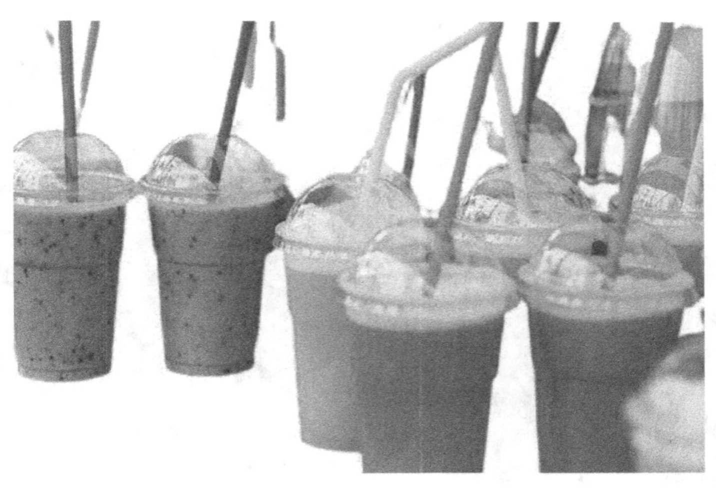

Dr. Mary Dixon

Copyright © 2023 by Dr. Mary Dixon

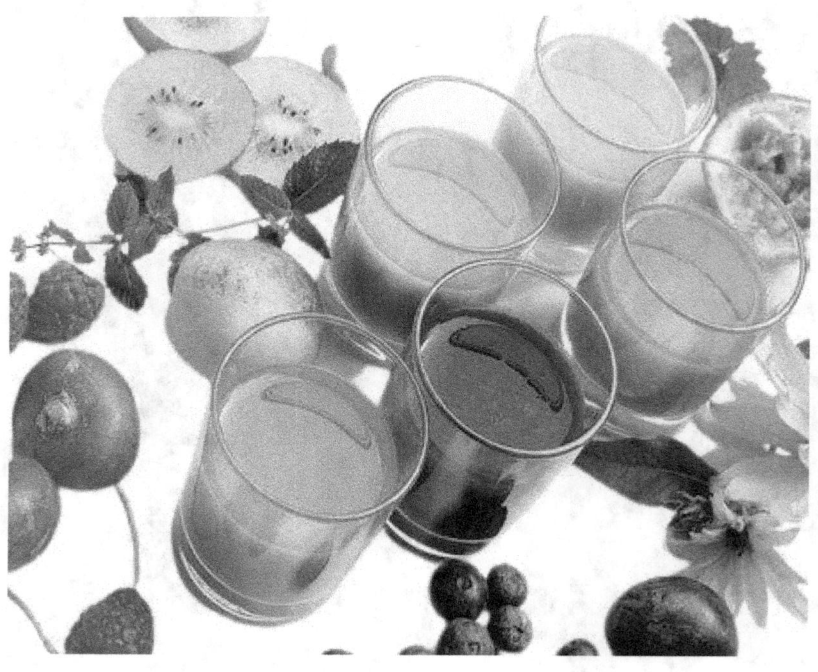

Table of Contents

INTRODUCTION 7

CHAPTER ONE 11

Thyroid Healing Explained.. 11

Types of Thyroids... 17

Causes of Thyroid 18

Symptoms of Thyroid 20

Prevention of Thyroid... 23

CHAPTER TWO 25

Thyroid Diet and Benefits.. 25

Benefits of a thyroid diet... 25

Foods to eat on a thyroid diet..................................... 27

Foods to avoid on a thyroid diet 28

How to Follow Thyroid Diet....................................... 30

7 Day Thyroid Meal Plan... 34

Day 1 34

Day 2 35

Day 4 38

Day 5 40

Day 6 41

Day 7 43

CHAPTER THREE 47

Smoothies for Thyroid Recipes 47

1. Green Mango Smoothie 47

2. Blueberry Banana Smoothie 48

3. Pineapple Turmeric Smoothie........................... 48

4. Spinach Berry Smoothie 49

5. Coconut Mango Smoothie 50

6. Cinnamon Apple Smoothie................................ 50

7. Peach Ginger Smoothie..................................... 51

8. Berry Beet Smoothie... 52

9. Chocolate Banana Smoothie 53

10. Matcha Smoothie 53

11. Orange Carrot Smoothie 54

12. Blueberry Kale Smoothie 55

13. Raspberry Coconut Smoothie 55

14. Pumpkin Pie Smoothie... 56

15. Mango Peach Smoothie 57

16. Cherry Almond Smoothie.. 57

17. Avocado Lime Smoothie 58

18. Strawberry Banana Smoothie 59

19. Chocolate Peanut Butter Smoothie 59

20. Peach Mango Smoothie 60

21. Blueberry Oatmeal Smoothie.................................... 61

22. Green Apple Smoothie... 61

23. Kiwi Pineapple Smoothie 62

24. Chocolate Cherry Smoothie...................................... 63

25. Turmeric Mango Smoothie.. 63

26. Coconut Pineapple Smoothie.................................... 64

27. Apple Cinnamon Smoothie....................................... 65

28. Strawberry Mango Smoothie 65

29. Pineapple Banana Smoothie 66

30. Vanilla Almond Smoothie 67

CONCLUSION... 69

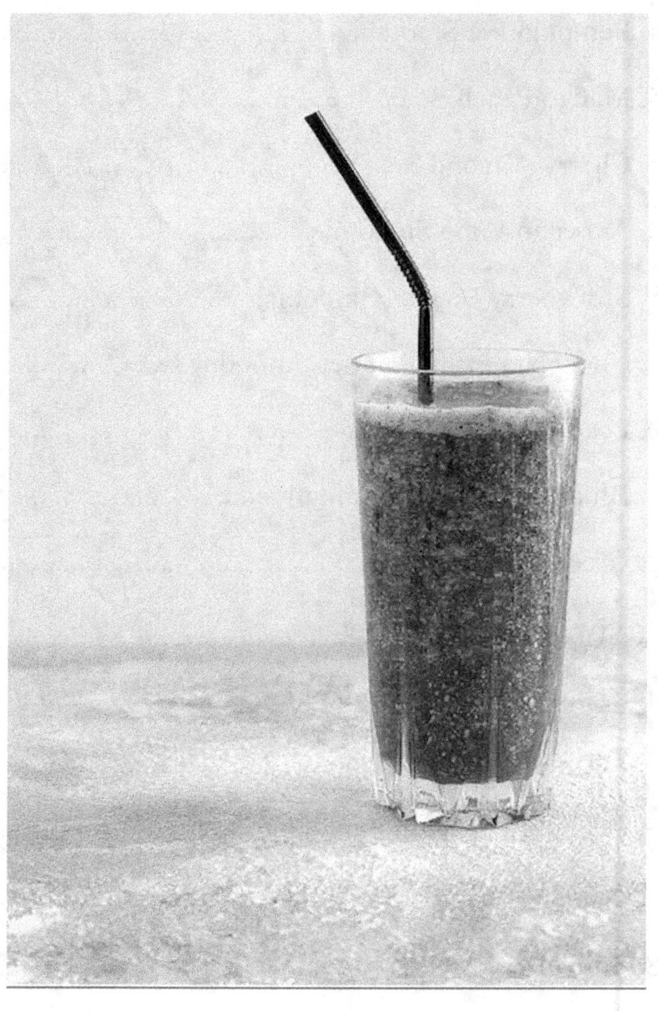

INTRODUCTION

Sophie had been struggling with thyroid problems for years. She had tried everything from medication to surgery, but nothing seemed to work. She was always feeling tired, gaining weight, and struggling with brain fog. It was a frustrating experience that left her feeling hopeless.

One day, while browsing online, Sophie came across a blog post about the benefits of smoothies for thyroid health. She was sceptical at first, but something about the article resonated with her, and she decided to give it a try.

Sophie began experimenting with different smoothie recipes, incorporating ingredients like kale, spinach, avocado, and berries. She made sure to include a mix of healthy fats, proteins, and carbohydrates to support her thyroid function.

To her surprise, Sophie noticed a significant improvement in her symptoms after just a few weeks of drinking smoothies regularly. Her energy levels increased, and she started losing weight without even trying.

Her brain fog lifted, and she felt more focused and alert.

Sophie was overjoyed. She had finally found a solution that worked for her. She continued to drink smoothies every day and even started sharing her recipes with friends who were struggling with similar health issues.

Thanks to the power of smoothies, Sophie was able to take control of her health and live the vibrant, energetic life she had always dreamed of.

The thyroid gland is an essential component of the endocrine system that plays a crucial role in regulating various bodily functions.

Located in the neck, just below the Adam's apple, the thyroid gland produces hormones that control metabolism, growth, and development.

These hormones are involved in almost every aspect of our daily lives, from controlling our heart rate and body temperature to affecting our mood and energy levels.

Thyroxine (T4) and triiodothyronine (T3) are the two main hormones produced by the thyroid gland. These hormones are made from iodine, a mineral that is found in many foods, including seafood, dairy products, and eggs.

The thyroid gland controls the production of these hormones by responding to signals from the pituitary gland, which is located in the brain.

When the thyroid gland is functioning correctly, it produces the right number of hormones to meet the body's needs. However, when it produces too much or too little of these hormones, it can lead to various health problems. Hyperthyroidism occurs when the thyroid gland produces too much thyroid hormone, while hypothyroidism occurs when it produces too little.

Hyperthyroidism can cause symptoms such as weight loss, nervousness, rapid heartbeat, and sweating. Hypothyroidism, on the other hand, can cause symptoms such as weight gain, fatigue, depression, and constipation. These symptoms can significantly impact a person's quality of life, and if left untreated, they can lead to more severe health problems.

In addition to hyperthyroidism and hypothyroidism, other thyroid-related conditions can also affect the gland's function. Thyroid nodules, for example, are small lumps that develop on the thyroid gland, and while they are usually benign, they can sometimes be cancerous. Thyroiditis, or inflammation of the thyroid gland, can also affect thyroid function, as can autoimmune disorders such as Graves' disease and Hashimoto's thyroiditis.

Diagnosing and treating thyroid conditions is essential to maintain overall health and well-being. Doctors can perform various tests to evaluate thyroid function, including blood tests to measure hormone levels, ultrasound to assess the size and appearance of the gland, and biopsy to examine tissue samples for abnormalities.

Treatment options depend on the specific condition and can include medication, surgery, or radioactive iodine therapy.

In conclusion, the thyroid gland is a critical component of the endocrine system that plays a crucial role in regulating many bodily functions.

When the thyroid gland is not functioning correctly, it can lead to a wide range of symptoms and health problems. Understanding the function of the thyroid gland and the various conditions that can affect it is essential for maintaining optimal health and well-being.

CHAPTER ONE

Thyroid Healing Explained

The thyroid, a little gland in the front of the neck that resembles a butterfly, is crucial for regulating hormone balance, metabolism, and energy production.

When the thyroid gland is not functioning properly, it can lead to a range of health problems, including weight gain or loss, fatigue, hair loss, depression, anxiety, and other issues.

Fortunately, there are many natural approaches to healing the thyroid and restoring optimal function. In this article, we will explore some of the most effective ways to support thyroid health, from dietary changes to lifestyle modifications and supplements.

Eat a Thyroid-Healthy Diet

One of the most important ways to support thyroid health is by following a diet that is rich in nutrients that are essential for thyroid function.

Some of the key nutrients include iodine, selenium, zinc, and iron.

A crucial mineral, iodine is required for the synthesis of thyroid hormones. Good dietary sources of iodine include seaweed, fish, dairy products, and iodized salt.

However, it is important not to overdo it with iodine supplements, as excessive intake can actually be harmful to the thyroid gland.

Selenium is another important nutrient that is essential for thyroid health. Good dietary sources of selenium include Brazil nuts, tuna, eggs, and sunflower seeds.

Zinc is important for the conversion of T4 to T3, the active form of thyroid hormone. Good dietary sources of zinc include oysters, beef, chicken, pumpkin seeds, and cashews.

Iron is also important for thyroid health, as it is needed for the production of thyroid hormones. Good dietary sources of iron include red meat, poultry, fish, beans, and spinach.

In addition to these key nutrients, it is important to eat a well-balanced diet that is rich in fruits, vegetables, whole grains, and lean protein. Avoid processed foods, sugar, and caffeine, which can disrupt thyroid function and contribute to inflammation in the body.

Reduce Stress

Stress is a major factor that can contribute to thyroid dysfunction. When the body is under chronic stress, it can lead to inflammation, hormonal imbalances, and a range of other health problems.

To support thyroid health, it is important to reduce stress levels through relaxation techniques such as meditation, yoga, or deep breathing exercises. Regular exercise is also beneficial for reducing stress and improving overall health.

Get Enough Sleep

Sleep is essential for overall health, and it is especially important for thyroid function. Lack of sleep can disrupt hormonal balance, increase inflammation, and contribute to a range of health problems.

To support thyroid health, aim for 7-8 hours of sleep per night. Make sure your bedtime routine includes relaxing activities like reading, taking a warm bath, and listening to soothing music.

Avoid screens and stimulating activities before bedtime, as these can disrupt sleep.

Supplement with Thyroid-Supportive Nutrients

In addition to dietary changes and lifestyle modifications, there are several supplements that can support thyroid health.

The following are some of the best supplements:

1. **Ashwagandha:** an adaptogenic plant that promotes thyroid health and stress reduction.

2. **Vitamin D:** a nutrient that is important for immune function and can help support thyroid health.

3. **Omega-3 fatty acids:** these healthy fats are anti-inflammatory and can help reduce inflammation in the body.

4. **B-complex vitamins:** these vitamins are important for energy production and can help support thyroid function.

It is crucial to speak with a healthcare practitioner before taking any supplements to be sure they are safe and suitable for your particular needs.

Address Underlying Health Issues

In some cases, thyroid dysfunction may be caused by underlying health issues such as autoimmune disorders, chronic inflammation, or nutrient deficiencies.

To support thyroid health, it is important to address these underlying issues through proper diagnosis and treatment.

Autoimmune disorders such as Hashimoto's thyroiditis and Graves' disease are common causes of thyroid dysfunction. In these circumstances, the thyroid gland is attacked by the immune system, which causes inflammation and damage.

Treatment may involve medications to regulate thyroid hormone levels and suppress the immune system, as well as dietary changes and lifestyle modifications to reduce inflammation and support immune function.

Chronic inflammation can also contribute to thyroid dysfunction. Addressing underlying inflammation through dietary changes, stress reduction, and supplements can help support thyroid health.

Finally, nutrient deficiencies such as low levels of iodine, selenium, or vitamin D can contribute to thyroid dysfunction. In these cases, supplementation or dietary changes may be necessary to restore optimal nutrient levels.

Seek Professional Help

If you are experiencing symptoms of thyroid dysfunction, it is important to seek professional help. A healthcare provider can perform a physical exam, order lab tests, and recommend treatment options that are tailored to your individual needs.

In some cases, medication may be necessary to regulate thyroid hormone levels and manage symptoms. However, many people are able to support thyroid health through natural approaches such as dietary changes, stress reduction, and supplements.

In conclusion, thyroid dysfunction is a common health problem that can cause a range of symptoms and health issues. By making dietary changes, reducing stress, getting enough sleep, supplementing with thyroid-supportive nutrients, addressing underlying health issues, and seeking professional help when needed, it is possible to support thyroid health and restore optimal function.

Types of Thyroids

1. **Hypothyroidism:** This is a condition in which the thyroid gland produces too little thyroid hormone, leading to a slower metabolism, weight gain, fatigue, and other symptoms.

2. **Hyperthyroidism:** This is a condition in which the thyroid gland produces too much thyroid hormone, leading to a faster metabolism, weight loss, anxiety, and other symptoms.

3. **Thyroiditis:** This is an inflammation of the thyroid gland that can cause temporary or permanent damage to the gland, leading to hypothyroidism or hyperthyroidism.

4. **Thyroid nodules:** These are lumps or growths that form on the thyroid gland. Although benign thyroid nodules are the majority, some can be cancerous.

5. **Thyroid cancer:** This is a type of cancer that develops in the cells of the thyroid gland. Papillary,

follicular, medullary, and anaplastic thyroid cancer are some of the several subtypes of thyroid cancer.

6. **Graves' disease:** This autoimmune condition causes hyperthyroidism when the immune system attacks the thyroid gland.

7. **Hashimoto's thyroiditis:** This is an autoimmune disorder in which the immune system attacks the thyroid gland, leading to hypothyroidism.

These are some of the most common types of thyroid conditions. The precise ailment and its severity will determine the available treatments.

Causes of Thyroid

1. **Autoimmune disorders:** In autoimmune disorders, the immune system attacks the thyroid gland, causing inflammation and damage that can lead to an underactive or overactive thyroid. The most common autoimmune disorder affecting the thyroid is Hashimoto's thyroiditis, which causes an underactive thyroid.

2. **Iodine deficiency:** Iodine is an essential nutrient that the thyroid needs to produce hormones. If you don't get enough iodine in your diet, the thyroid may not be able to produce enough hormones, leading to an underactive thyroid.

3. **Radiation therapy:** Radiation therapy to the head and neck can damage the thyroid gland, leading to an underactive thyroid.

4. **Medications:** Certain medications, such as lithium, interferon alpha, and amiodarone, can interfere with thyroid function and cause an underactive or overactive thyroid.

5. **Genetics:** Thyroid disorders can run in families, suggesting that genetic factors may play a role in their development.

6. **Inflammation:** Inflammation of the thyroid gland, known as thyroiditis, can cause temporary thyroid dysfunction. This can be triggered by infections, medications, or other factors.

7. **Pituitary gland disorders:** The pituitary gland produces thyroid-stimulating hormone (TSH), which signals the thyroid to produce hormones. If the pituitary gland isn't working correctly, it can lead to an underactive thyroid.

Overall, there are several potential causes of thyroid disorders, including autoimmune disorders, iodine deficiency, radiation therapy, medications, genetics, inflammation, and pituitary gland disorders.

If you're experiencing symptoms of a thyroid disorder, it's important to talk to your healthcare provider to determine the underlying cause and develop an appropriate treatment plan.

Symptoms of Thyroid

1. **Fatigue:** Feeling tired and lacking energy is a common symptom of an underactive thyroid (hypothyroidism). This is because thyroid hormone plays a key role in regulating the body's energy levels.

2. **Weight changes:** Both hyperthyroidism and hypothyroidism can cause changes in weight.

People with hypothyroidism may gain weight due to a slowed metabolism, while those with hyperthyroidism may lose weight due to an increased metabolism.

3. **Hair loss:** Thyroid disorders can lead to hair loss, especially on the scalp and eyebrows. This is because thyroid hormone helps regulate hair growth.

4. **Mood changes:** Thyroid hormone can affect mood, and people with thyroid disorders may experience anxiety, depression, irritability, or other mood changes.

5. **Skin changes:** Dry skin, itching, and other skin changes can occur due to a thyroid disorder.

6. **Menstrual irregularities:** Thyroid hormone helps regulate the menstrual cycle, and thyroid disorders can cause menstrual irregularities such as heavy or irregular periods.

7. **Muscle weakness:** People with hypothyroidism may experience muscle weakness, while those with

hyperthyroidism may experience muscle tremors or weakness.

8. **Heart rate changes:** Hyperthyroidism can cause a rapid or irregular heartbeat, while hypothyroidism can cause a slow heartbeat.

9. **Digestive issues:** Constipation and other digestive issues can occur due to a thyroid disorder.

10. **Heat or cold intolerance:** People with hypothyroidism may feel cold all the time, while those with hyperthyroidism may feel hot and sweaty.

It's important to note that these symptoms can vary depending on the type and severity of the thyroid disorder, and some people may experience no symptoms at all.

If you suspect you may have a thyroid disorder, it's important to talk to your healthcare provider for proper diagnosis and treatment.

Prevention of Thyroid

1. **Iodine-rich Diet:** Iodine is an essential nutrient for thyroid function, and a deficiency in iodine can cause hypothyroidism. You can prevent iodine deficiency by consuming iodine-rich foods such as seaweed, fish, dairy products, and iodized salt.

2. **Selenium-rich Diet:** Selenium is another essential nutrient for thyroid function, and it helps convert the thyroid hormone T4 to its active form, T3. Consuming foods such as Brazil nuts, fish, and eggs can help ensure adequate selenium intake.

3. **Avoid Goitrogens:** Goitrogens are substances that interfere with thyroid function and can cause goitre, an enlarged thyroid gland. Some foods that contain goitrogens include soy products, cruciferous vegetables (such as broccoli and cauliflower), and certain fruits. While these foods can still be consumed in moderation, it is important to avoid excessive consumption.

4. **Manage Stress:** Chronic stress can negatively affect thyroid function by increasing cortisol levels, which can interfere with thyroid hormone production. Practicing stress-management techniques such as meditation, yoga, or deep breathing can help promote thyroid health.

5. **Regular Check-ups:** Regular thyroid function testing can help detect any potential thyroid problems early on. It is recommended that individuals over the age of 35 get a thyroid function test every five years.

In conclusion, while some thyroid problems cannot be prevented, promoting a healthy lifestyle through a balanced diet, stress management, and regular check-ups can help reduce the risk of thyroid disorders and promote overall thyroid health.

CHAPTER TWO

Thyroid Diet and Benefits

What is the thyroid diet?

The thyroid diet is a way of eating that focuses on nutrients that support thyroid function. The diet emphasizes nutrient-dense, whole foods that are rich in vitamins and minerals, as well as specific foods that are beneficial for thyroid health. The diet also recommends avoiding certain foods that can interfere with thyroid function.

Benefits of a thyroid diet

1. **Helps regulate thyroid function:** The thyroid diet includes foods that are rich in iodine, selenium, and zinc, which are essential for healthy thyroid function. These nutrients help the thyroid produce hormones that regulate metabolism, energy levels, and body weight.

2. **Promotes weight loss:** Thyroid conditions can often lead to weight gain, and losing weight can be difficult. The thyroid diet encourages eating nutrient-

dense, whole foods, and avoiding processed foods and refined sugars. This approach can help promote weight loss and improve overall health.

3. **Reduces inflammation:** Inflammation can interfere with thyroid function, and a diet that is high in anti-inflammatory foods can help reduce inflammation in the body. The thyroid diet includes foods like leafy greens, fatty fish, and berries, which are all known for their anti-inflammatory properties.

4. **Improves energy levels:** Fatigue is a common symptom of thyroid conditions, and the thyroid diet includes foods that are rich in nutrients that can boost energy levels. Foods like whole grains, lean protein, and healthy fats can help provide sustained energy throughout the day.

5. **Supports mental health:** Thyroid conditions can also lead to depression and anxiety, and a diet that is rich in nutrients like omega-3 fatty acids, vitamin D, and magnesium can help support mental health. These nutrients are found in foods like fatty fish, eggs, and leafy greens.

Foods to eat on a thyroid diet

The following foods are recommended for a thyroid-friendly diet:

1. **Sea vegetables:** Sea vegetables like kelp and nori are rich in iodine, which is essential for thyroid function.

2. **Lean protein:** Lean protein sources like chicken, turkey, and fish are rich in selenium, which is important for healthy thyroid function.

3. **Whole grains:** Whole grains like brown rice and quinoa provide sustained energy and are rich in B vitamins, which are essential for thyroid health.

4. **Fruits and vegetables:** Fruits and vegetables are rich in antioxidants and other nutrients that support thyroid health. In particular, leafy greens like spinach and kale are advantageous.

5. **Healthy fats:** Healthy fats like avocados, nuts, and seeds are important for overall health and can help support thyroid function.

Foods to avoid on a thyroid diet

The following foods are best avoided on a thyroid-friendly diet:

1. Soy products: Soy can interfere with thyroid function, especially in people with an underactive thyroid.

2. Processed foods: Processed foods are often high in refined sugars and other additives that can interfere with thyroid function.

3. Gluten: Some people with thyroid conditions may be sensitive to gluten, and avoiding gluten can help reduce inflammation in the body.

4. Alcohol and caffeine: Alcohol and caffeine can interfere with thyroid function and should be consumed in moderation.

A thyroid-friendly diet is a way of eating that emphasizes nutrient-dense, whole foods and includes specific foods that support thyroid function.

This approach can help regulate thyroid function, promote weight loss, reduce inflammation, improve energy levels, and support mental health.

By focusing on foods that are rich in iodine, selenium, zinc, and other nutrients, and avoiding foods that can interfere with thyroid function, individuals can optimize their thyroid health and overall well-being.

While adopting a thyroid-friendly diet can be beneficial for those with thyroid conditions, it's important to note that it is not a substitute for medical treatment.

Anyone with a thyroid condition should work closely with their healthcare provider to develop a treatment plan that includes medication and lifestyle changes.

In addition to following a thyroid-friendly diet, there are other lifestyle changes that individuals with thyroid conditions can make to support their health.

These include getting enough sleep, managing stress, and engaging in regular exercise. All of these lifestyle factors can impact thyroid function and overall health.

In conclusion, a thyroid-friendly diet is a healthy way of eating that can support thyroid function and overall health. By focusing on nutrient-dense, whole foods and avoiding foods that can interfere with thyroid function, individuals can optimize their thyroid health and improve their overall well-being. Along with other lifestyle changes, a thyroid-friendly diet can be an important part of a comprehensive approach to managing thyroid conditions.

How to Follow Thyroid Diet

A thyroid diet is a way of eating that focuses on foods that can support the health of the thyroid gland. It's important to note that a thyroid diet is not a cure for thyroid problems, but it can help manage symptoms and improve overall health. **Here are some tips on how to follow a thyroid diet:**

Focus on nutrient-dense foods:

Nutrient-dense foods are those that are high in vitamins, minerals, and other nutrients that are important for overall health.

These include:

1. **Fruits and vegetables:** Aim to eat a variety of colourful fruits and vegetables to get a wide range of nutrients.

2. **Whole grains:** Choose whole grains over refined grains, such as brown rice, quinoa, and whole wheat bread.

3. **Lean proteins:** Choose lean proteins such as chicken, fish, and tofu to help support muscle growth and repair.

4. **Healthy fats:** Include healthy fats such as olive oil, avocados, and nuts in your diet to help support brain function and hormone production.

Avoid goitrogenic foods:

Goitrogenic foods are those that can interfere with the function of the thyroid gland. **These include:**

1. **Cruciferous vegetables:** Vegetables such as broccoli, cauliflower, and kale contain compounds that can interfere with thyroid function.

2. **Soy:** Soy contains compounds that can interfere with the absorption of iodine, which is essential for thyroid function.

3. **Gluten:** Some people with thyroid problems also have gluten sensitivity, so it's important to consider eliminating gluten from your diet if you experience symptoms such as bloating, gas, and diarrhoea.

Eat foods rich in iodine:

The creation of thyroid hormones requires iodine. **Iodine-rich food items include:**

1. **Seafood:** Seafood such as shrimp, salmon, and tuna are excellent sources of iodine.

2. **Seaweed:** Seaweed is a rich source of iodine and can be incorporated into soups, salads, and stir-fries.

3. **Dairy products:** Milk and cheese are examples of dairy items that are excellent suppliers of iodine.

Consider selenium:

A mineral that is crucial for thyroid health is selenium. **Among the foods high in selenium are:**

1. **Brazil nuts:** One of the best sources of selenium is Brazil nuts.

2. **Fish:** Fish such as tuna, halibut, and sardines are also good sources of selenium.

3. **Eggs:** Eggs are another good source of selenium.

Limit processed foods:

Processed foods are often high in sugar, salt, and unhealthy fats, which can contribute to inflammation and negatively impact thyroid function. Aim to consume less processed foods and more complete, nutrient-dense foods.

Following a thyroid diet can be a helpful way to support the health of your thyroid gland.

By focusing on nutrient-dense foods, avoiding goitrogenic foods, and incorporating iodine and selenium-rich foods into your diet, you can help manage symptoms and improve overall health.

7 Day Thyroid Meal Plan

Day 1

Breakfast:

Quinoa Porridge with Blueberries and Walnuts

1. Cook 1/2 cup of quinoa in 1 cup of almond milk until tender.

2. Add 1 tbsp of maple syrup, 1/4 tsp of cinnamon, 1/4 tsp of vanilla extract, and a pinch of salt to the porridge.

3. Top with 1/2 cup of blueberries and 2 tbsp of chopped walnuts.

Lunch:

Avocado and Chickpea Salad

1. In a bowl, mix together 1 can of drained and rinsed chickpeas, 1 diced avocado, 1/4 cup of diced red onion, 1/4 cup of diced cucumber, and 1/4 cup of chopped fresh cilantro.

2. Drizzle with 1 tbsp of olive oil and 1 tbsp of lemon juice.

Dinner:

Grilled Salmon with Roasted Vegetables

1. Preheat oven to 400°F. Cut 1 sweet potato and 1 bell pepper into 1-inch pieces.

2. Toss the vegetables with 1 tbsp of olive oil and a pinch of salt. 20–25 minutes, or until soft, in the oven.

3. Season 1 salmon fillet with 1/2 tsp of paprika, 1/4 tsp of garlic powder, and a pinch of salt. Grill for 6-8 minutes on each side, or until cooked through.

Day 2

Breakfast:

Greek Yogurt with Berries and Granola

1. Mix 1 cup of Greek yogurt with 1/2 cup of mixed berries and 1/4 cup of granola.

Lunch:

Lentil Soup with Mixed Vegetables

2. In a pot, sauté 1 chopped onion and 2 minced garlic cloves in 1 tbsp of olive oil until soft.

3. Add 1 cup of diced mixed vegetables, 1 can of drained and rinsed lentils, and 4 cups of vegetable broth. Simmer for 20 minutes.

4. Season with 1 tsp of cumin, 1/2 tsp of coriander, and a pinch of salt.

Dinner:

Baked Chicken with Cauliflower Rice

1. Preheat oven to 375°F. Season 1 chicken breast with 1/2 tsp of dried oregano, 1/4 tsp of garlic powder, and a pinch of salt.

2. Bake for 25 to 30 minutes, or until thoroughly done.

3. Serve with 1 cup of cauliflower rice, seasoned with 1 tbsp of coconut oil and a pinch of salt.

Day 3

Breakfast:

Green Smoothie Bowl

1. Blend 1 cup of unsweetened almond milk, 1 frozen banana, 1 cup of spinach, and 1/2 cup of frozen pineapple in a blender until smooth.

2. Top with 1/4 cup of sliced strawberries, 1 tbsp of chia seeds, and 1 tbsp of shredded coconut.

Lunch:

Quinoa and Black Bean Salad

1. Cook 1 cup of quinoa in 2 cups of vegetable broth until tender.

2. Mix together the cooked quinoa, 1 can of drained and rinsed black beans, 1/2 cup of diced red onion, 1/2 cup of diced tomato, and 1/4 cup of chopped fresh cilantro.

3. Drizzle with 1 tbsp of olive oil and 1 tbsp of lime juice.

Dinner:

Roasted Vegetable and Chickpea Bowl

1. Preheat oven to 400°F. Cut 1 sweet potato, 1 red bell pepper, and 1 zucchini into 1-inch pieces.

2. Toss the vegetables with 1 tbsp of olive oil and a pinch of salt. 20–25 minutes, or until soft, in the oven.

3. In a pan, sauté 1 can of drained and rinsed chickpeas with 1 tsp of cumin, 1/2 tsp of coriander, and a pinch of salt for 5-7 minutes, or until heated through.

4. Serve the chickpeas and roasted vegetables on top of quinoa that has been cooked.

Day 4

Breakfast:

Gluten-Free Banana Pancakes

1. In a blender, blend together 2 ripe bananas, 2 eggs, 1/2 cup of almond flour, 1 tsp of baking powder, and a pinch of salt until smooth.

2. Heat a non-stick pan over medium heat. Pour 1/4 cup of batter onto the pan and cook for 2-3 minutes on each side, or until golden brown.

3. Serve with 1/2 cup of fresh berries.

Lunch:

Tuna Salad Lettuce Wraps

1. Mix together 1 can of drained and flaked tuna, 1/4 cup of diced celery, 1/4 cup of diced red onion, 1 tbsp of mayonnaise, and a pinch of salt.

2. Spoon the tuna salad onto 4 large lettuce leaves and wrap.

Dinner:

Grilled Chicken and Vegetable Kebabs

1. Preheat grill to medium-high heat. Cut 1 chicken breast, 1 red bell pepper, 1 yellow squash, and 1 zucchini into bite-sized pieces.

2. Thread the chicken and vegetables onto skewers. Brush with 1 tbsp of olive oil and season with 1 tsp of dried oregano and a pinch of salt.

3. Grill food for 10 to 12 minutes, or until well done.

Day 5

Breakfast:

Apple Cinnamon Oatmeal

1. In a pot, bring 1 cup of water and 1/2 cup of almond milk to a boil.

2. Add 1/2 cup of rolled oats, 1 diced apple, 1 tsp of cinnamon, and a pinch of salt. Cook the oats for 5-7 minutes, or until they are soft.

3. Top with 1 tbsp of almond butter and a drizzle of maple syrup.

Lunch:

Roasted Vegetable and Quinoa Bowl

1. Preheat oven to 400°F. Cut 1 sweet potato, 1 red bell pepper, and 1 zucchini into 1-inch pieces.

2. Toss the vegetables with 1 tbsp of olive oil and a pinch of salt. 20–25 minutes, or until soft, in the oven.

3. Serve the roasted vegetables on top of quinoa that has been cooked.

Dinner:

Baked Salmon with Asparagus

1. Preheat oven to 375°F. Season 1 salmon fillet with 1/2 tsp of dried dill, 1/4 tsp of garlic powder, and a pinch of salt.

2. Bake for 20-25 minutes, or until cooked through.

3. Serve with 1 cup of roasted asparagus, seasoned with 1 tbsp of olive oil and a pinch of salt.

Day 6

Breakfast:

Blueberry Chia Pudding

1. In a jar, mix together 1 cup of unsweetened almond milk, 1/2 cup of chia seeds, 1 tbsp of maple syrup, and 1/2 tsp of vanilla extract.

2. Stir in 1/2 cup of fresh blueberries. Refrigerate overnight or for at least two hours.

Lunch:

Turkey and Avocado Lettuce Wraps

1. Fill 4 large lettuce leaves with 4 slices of deli turkey, 1/2 sliced avocado, and 1/4 cup of diced tomato.

Dinner:

Beef and Vegetable Stir-Fry

2. In a pan, heat 1 tbsp of sesame oil over high heat. Add 1 lb of thinly sliced beef and cook for 2-3 minutes, or until browned.

3. Add 1 sliced onion, 1 sliced bell pepper, and 1 cup of sliced mushrooms. Cook the vegetables for a further 2 to 3 minutes, or until they are soft.

4. In a bowl, mix together 1 tbsp of corn-starch and 2 tbsp of soy sauce. Pour over the beef and vegetables and cook for 1-2 minutes, or until the sauce thickens.

5. Over cooked brown rice, if desired.

Day 7

Breakfast:

Green Smoothie

- In a blender, blend together 1 banana, 1/2 cup of frozen mango, 1/2 cup of fresh spinach, 1 tbsp of almond butter, and 1 cup of unsweetened almond milk.

Lunch:

Greek Salad

- Toss together 2 cups of mixed greens, 1/4 cup of sliced cucumber, 1/4 cup of sliced cherry tomatoes, 1/4 cup of sliced red onion, 1/4 cup of crumbled feta cheese, and 2 tbsp of Greek vinaigrette.

Dinner:

Lemon Garlic Shrimp with Broccoli

1. 1 tablespoon of olive oil is heated in a pan over medium-high heat. Add 1 lb of peeled and deveined shrimp and cook for 2-3 minutes, or until pink.

2. Add 1 cup of chopped broccoli and cook for an additional 2-3 minutes, or until the broccoli is tender.

3. In a small bowl, whisk together 1 minced garlic clove, 1 tbsp of lemon juice, and a pinch of salt. Pour over the shrimp and broccoli and cook for 1-2 minutes, or until heated through.

4. Serve over a bed of brown rice or cooked quinoa.

Snack Ideas:

- Apple slices with almond butter

- Carrot sticks with hummus

- Greek yogurt with berries and granola

- Roasted chickpeas

- Hard boiled eggs

- Mixed nuts and dried fruit

Note: This meal plan is designed to provide general ideas and inspiration for a thyroid-friendly diet.

It is important to consult with a healthcare provider or registered dietitian to determine an appropriate meal plan that meets individual nutritional needs and health goals.

Additionally, some individuals may have specific dietary restrictions or food allergies that should be taken into consideration when planning meals.

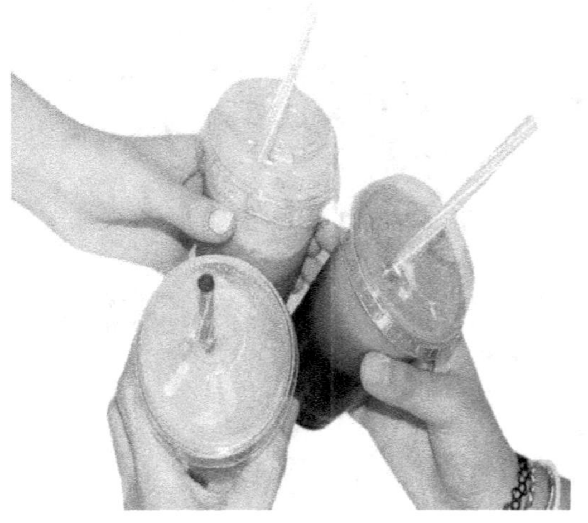

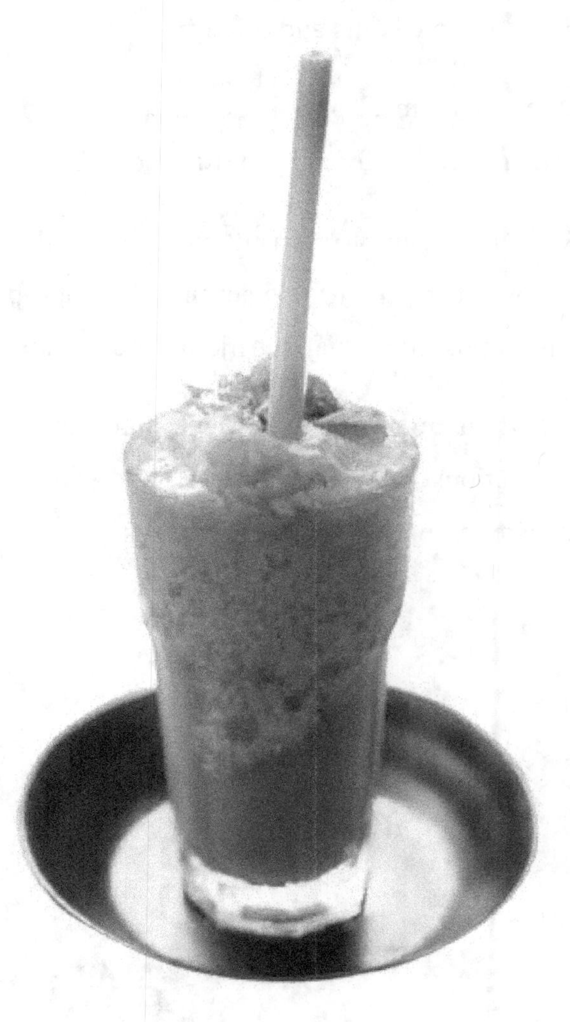

CHAPTER THREE

Smoothies for Thyroid Recipes

The thyroid gland is a crucial part of the endocrine system and plays an essential role in regulating metabolism and hormonal balance.

Smoothies can be an excellent way to support thyroid health by incorporating nutrient-dense ingredients that are rich in vitamins, minerals, and antioxidants.

Here are 30 thyroid-friendly smoothie recipes that are easy to make and delicious.

1. Green Mango Smoothie

Ingredients:

- 1 cup spinach

- 1 cup frozen mango chunks

- 1/2 avocado

- 1 tbsp chia seeds

- 1/2 cup unsweetened almond milk

Instructions:

1. Blend all ingredients until smooth. Enjoy!

Cooking time: 5 minutes

2. Blueberry Banana Smoothie

Ingredients:

- 1 banana
- 1 cup frozen blueberries
- 1 tbsp hemp seeds
- 1/2 cup plain Greek yogurt
- 1/2 cup unsweetened almond milk

Instructions:

1. Blend all ingredients until smooth. Enjoy!

Cooking time: 5 minutes

3. Pineapple Turmeric Smoothie

Ingredients:

- 1 cup frozen pineapple chunks

- 1/2 banana

- 1/2 tsp ground turmeric

- 1 tbsp fresh ginger

- 1/2 cup unsweetened coconut milk

Instructions:

1. Blend all ingredients until smooth. Enjoy!

Cooking time: 5 minutes

4. Spinach Berry Smoothie

Ingredients:

- 1 cup spinach

- 1/2 cup frozen mixed berries

- 1/2 banana

- 1 tbsp almond butter

- 1/2 cup unsweetened almond milk

Instructions:

1. Blend all ingredients until smooth. Enjoy!

Cooking time: 5 minutes

5. Coconut Mango Smoothie

Ingredients:

- 1 cup frozen mango chunks

- 1/2 cup plain Greek yogurt

- 1/2 cup unsweetened coconut milk

- 1 tbsp shredded coconut

- 1/2 tsp vanilla extract

Instructions:

1. Blend all ingredients until smooth. Enjoy!

Cooking time: 5 minutes

6. Cinnamon Apple Smoothie

Ingredients:

- 1 apple, cored and chopped

- 1/2 banana

- 1 tsp ground cinnamon

- 1/2 cup unsweetened almond milk

- 1 tbsp honey

Instructions:

1. Blend all ingredients until smooth. Enjoy!

Cooking time: 5 minutes

7. Peach Ginger Smoothie

Ingredients:

- 1 cup frozen peaches

- 1 tbsp fresh ginger

- 1/2 cup plain Greek yogurt

- 1/2 cup unsweetened almond milk

- 1 tsp honey

Instructions:

1.   Blend all ingredients until smooth. Enjoy!

Cooking time: 5 minutes

8. Berry Beet Smoothie

Ingredients:

- 1 cup frozen mixed berries

- 1/2 cooked beet, peeled and chopped

- 1/2 banana

- 1/2 cup unsweetened almond milk

- 1 tbsp honey

Instructions:

1.   Blend all ingredients until smooth. Enjoy!

Cooking time: 5 minutes

9. Chocolate Banana Smoothie

Ingredients:

- 1 banana

- 1 tbsp cacao powder

- 1 tbsp almond butter

- 1/2 cup unsweetened almond milk

- 1 tsp honey

Instructions:

1. Blend all ingredients until smooth. Enjoy!

Cooking time: 5 minutes

10. Matcha Smoothie

Ingredients:

- 1 tsp matcha powder

- 1/2 banana

- 1/2 cup plain Greek yogurt

- 1/2 cup unsweetened almond milk

- 1 tsp honey

Instructions:

1. Blend all ingredients until smooth. Enjoy!

11. Orange Carrot Smoothie

Ingredients:

- 1 orange, peeled and segmented

- 1 medium carrot, peeled and chopped

- 1/2 cup unsweetened coconut milk

- 1 tbsp honey

- 1/2 tsp vanilla extract

Instructions:

1. Blend all ingredients until smooth. Enjoy!

Cooking time: 5 minutes

12. Blueberry Kale Smoothie

Ingredients:

- 1 cup kale

- 1 cup frozen blueberries

- 1/2 banana

- 1/2 cup unsweetened almond milk

- 1 tbsp honey

Instructions:

1. Blend all ingredients until smooth. Enjoy!

Cooking time: 5 minutes

13. Raspberry Coconut Smoothie

Ingredients:

- 1 cup frozen raspberries

- 1/2 cup plain Greek yogurt

- 1/2 cup unsweetened coconut milk

- 1 tbsp shredded coconut

- 1 tsp honey

Instructions:

1. Blend all ingredients until smooth. Enjoy!

Cooking time: 5 minutes

14. Pumpkin Pie Smoothie

Ingredients:

- 1/2 cup canned pumpkin puree

- 1/2 banana

- 1 tsp pumpkin pie spice

- 1/2 cup unsweetened almond milk

- 1 tbsp honey

Instructions:

1. Blend all ingredients until smooth. Enjoy!

Cooking time: 5 minutes

15. Mango Peach Smoothie

Ingredients:

- 1 cup frozen mango chunks

- 1 cup frozen peaches

- 1/2 cup plain Greek yogurt

- 1/2 cup unsweetened almond milk

- 1 tsp honey

Instructions:

1. Blend all ingredients until smooth. Enjoy!

Cooking time: 5 minutes

16. Cherry Almond Smoothie

Ingredients:

- 1 cup frozen cherries

- 1 tbsp almond butter

- 1/2 cup plain Greek yogurt

- 1/2 cup unsweetened almond milk

- 1 tsp honey

Instructions:

1. Blend all ingredients until smooth. Enjoy!

Cooking time: 5 minutes

17. Avocado Lime Smoothie

Ingredients:

- 1/2 avocado

- 1 lime, juiced

- 1 cup spinach

- 1/2 cup unsweetened coconut milk

- 1 tbsp honey

Instructions:

1. Blend all ingredients until smooth. Enjoy!

Cooking time: 5 minutes

18. Strawberry Banana Smoothie

Ingredients:

- 1 banana

- 1 cup frozen strawberries

- 1/2 cup plain Greek yogurt

- 1/2 cup unsweetened almond milk

- 1 tsp honey

Instructions:

1. Blend all ingredients until smooth. Enjoy!

Cooking time: 5 minutes

19. Chocolate Peanut Butter Smoothie

Ingredients:

- 1 banana

- 1 tbsp cacao powder

- 1 tbsp peanut butter

- 1/2 cup unsweetened almond milk

- 1 tsp honey

Instructions:

1. Blend all ingredients until smooth. Enjoy!

Cooking time: 5 minutes

20. Peach Mango Smoothie

Ingredients:

- 1 cup frozen peaches

- 1 cup frozen mango chunks

- 1/2 cup plain Greek yogurt

- 1/2 cup unsweetened almond milk

- 1 tsp honey

Instructions:

1. Blend all ingredients until smooth. Enjoy!

Cooking time: 5 minutes

21. Blueberry Oatmeal Smoothie

Ingredients:

- 1/2 cup rolled oats

- 1 cup frozen blueberries

- 1/2 banana

- 1/2 cup unsweetened almond milk

- 1 tsp honey

Instructions:

1. Blend all ingredients until smooth. Enjoy!

Cooking time: 5 minutes

22. Green Apple Smoothie

Ingredients:

- 1 green apple, cored and chopped

- 1/2 banana

- 1 cup spinach

- 1/2 cup unsweetened almond milk

- 1 tsp honey

Instructions:

1. Blend all ingredients until smooth. Enjoy!

Cooking time: 5 minutes

23. Kiwi Pineapple Smoothie

Ingredients:

- 2 kiwis, peeled and chopped

- 1 cup frozen pineapple chunks

- 1/2 cup plain Greek yogurt

- 1/2 cup unsweetened coconut milk

- 1 tsp honey

Instructions:

1. Blend all ingredients until smooth. Enjoy!

Cooking time: 5 minutes

24. Chocolate Cherry Smoothie

Ingredients:

- 1 cup frozen cherries

- 1 tbsp cacao powder

- 1/2 cup plain Greek yogurt

- 1/2 cup unsweetened almond milk

- 1 tsp honey

Instructions:

1. Blend all ingredients until smooth. Enjoy!

Cooking time: 5 minutes

25. Turmeric Mango Smoothie

Ingredients:

- 1 cup frozen mango chunks

- 1/2 tsp turmeric powder

- 1/2 cup plain Greek yogurt

* 1/2 cup unsweetened almond milk

* 1 tsp honey

Instructions:

1.   Blend all ingredients until smooth. Enjoy!

Cooking time: 5 minutes

26. Coconut Pineapple Smoothie

Ingredients:

* 1 cup frozen pineapple chunks

* 1/2 cup unsweetened coconut milk

* 1/2 cup plain Greek yogurt

* 1 tbsp shredded coconut

* 1 tsp honey

Instructions:

Blend all ingredients until smooth. Enjoy!

Cooking time: 5 minutes

27. Apple Cinnamon Smoothie

Ingredients:

- 1 apple, cored and chopped

- 1/2 tsp cinnamon

- 1 cup spinach

- 1/2 cup unsweetened almond milk

- 1 tsp honey

Instructions:

Blend all ingredients until smooth. Enjoy!

Cooking time: 5 minutes

28. Strawberry Mango Smoothie

Ingredients:

- 1 cup frozen mango chunks

- 1 cup frozen strawberries

- 1/2 cup plain Greek yogurt

- 1/2 cup unsweetened almond milk

- 1 tsp honey

Instructions:

1. Blend all ingredients until smooth. Enjoy!

Cooking time: 5 minutes

29. Pineapple Banana Smoothie

Ingredients:

- 1 banana

- 1 cup frozen pineapple chunks

- 1/2 cup plain Greek yogurt

- 1/2 cup unsweetened coconut milk

- 1 tsp honey

Instructions:

1. Blend all ingredients until smooth. Enjoy!

Cooking time: 5 minutes

30. Vanilla Almond Smoothie

Ingredients:

- 1/2 cup plain Greek yogurt

- 1/2 cup unsweetened almond milk

- 1 tsp vanilla extract

- 1 tbsp almond butter

- 1 tsp honey

Instructions:

1. Blend all ingredients until smooth. Enjoy!

Cooking time: 5 minutes

These are 30 delicious and healthy smoothie recipes that are perfect for thyroid health.

With a variety of ingredients and flavours, you'll never get bored of enjoying these smoothies. Plus, they're easy to make and can be whipped up in just 5 minutes!

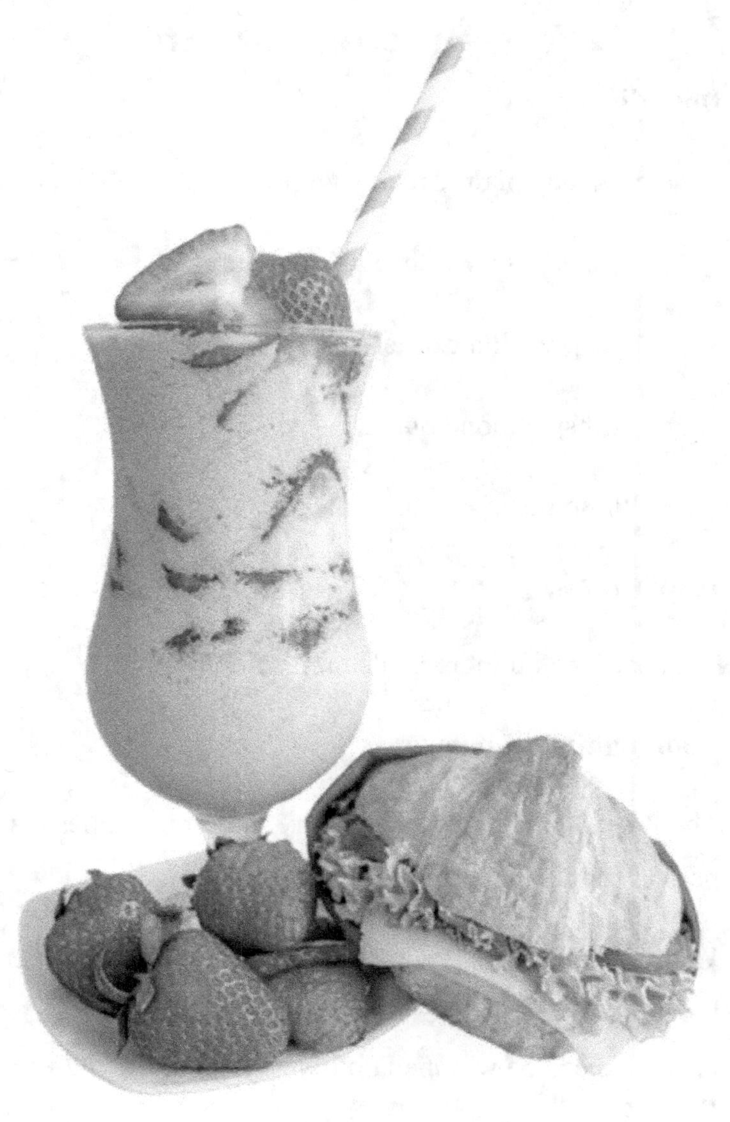

CONCLUSION

In conclusion, smoothies can be a great addition to the diet of individuals with thyroid disorders. By incorporating specific ingredients that are known to support thyroid function, such as fruits and vegetables rich in vitamins and minerals, healthy fats, and protein sources, smoothies can help maintain optimal thyroid hormone levels and support overall health and well-being.

Some of the best ingredients to include in a smoothie for thyroid health include leafy greens like spinach and kale, which are rich in vitamins and minerals like magnesium and vitamin A, both of which are essential for thyroid health. Additionally, fruits like berries and bananas can provide antioxidants and fibre, which can help reduce inflammation and support digestion.

Healthy fats like avocado, coconut oil, and nuts can also be excellent additions to a thyroid-friendly smoothie. These fats are important for hormone synthesis and can help keep blood sugar levels stable, which is crucial for individuals with thyroid disorders.

Protein sources like Greek yogurt, whey protein powder, or nut butter can also be beneficial for thyroid health. Protein is essential for building and repairing tissues, and it can also help regulate hormone production and balance blood sugar levels.

Overall, smoothies can be a convenient and easy way to get important nutrients that support thyroid health, especially for individuals who have difficulty eating a varied and balanced diet. However, it's important to note that smoothies should not be relied on as the sole source of nutrition and should be consumed in conjunction with a well-rounded diet.

It's also important to consult with a healthcare provider before incorporating smoothies into your diet, especially if you are taking thyroid medication or have other health conditions.

In conclusion, smoothies can be a delicious and effective way to support thyroid health. By incorporating a variety of thyroid-supporting ingredients like leafy greens, fruits, healthy fats, and protein sources, individuals with thyroid disorders can help maintain optimal thyroid function and promote overall health and wellness.